STACY C. GLASS

Hashimoto's Diet Recipes Cookbook

Healing Thyroid, Hypothyroidism, Easy No Stress Meal Plan, Autoimmune Health Protocol For Getting Your Life Back

Contents

Introduction

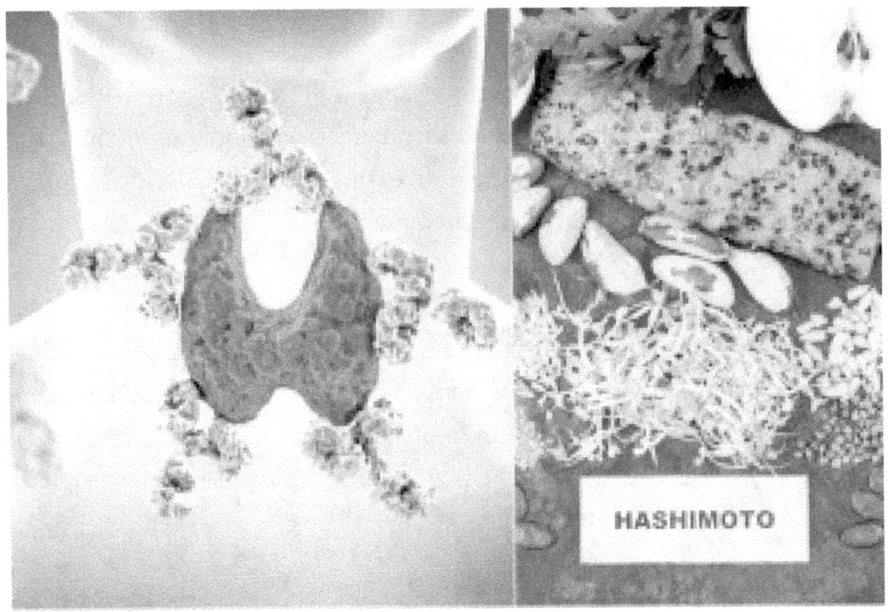

A Personal Journey

As I sit down to write this, I am reminded of times when my health felt like a puzzle with missing pieces. The weariness, the cognitive fog, the unexpected weight gain—it all seems insurmountable. But suddenly, like a beacon of hope, I came upon the concept of Hashimoto's diet. I had no idea it would become my lifeline—a way to recover and reclaim my vitality.

The diagnosis

The doctor's words rang in my head: "You have Hashimoto's thyroiditis." It was simultaneously a relief and a challenge. Finally, a term for the invisible force that is doing havoc on my body. Hashimoto's is an autoimmune disorder in which my immune system erroneously attacks my thyroid gland. Suddenly, my symptoms made sense: slow metabolism, hair loss, and mood swings. However, understanding the problem was only the first step.

The Turning Point

I started on a quest that would change my relationship with food. Hashimoto's diet was more than just what I ate; it was about nourishing my body, boosting my immune system, and easing the inflammation that had taken hold of me. Here's how it changed my life.

1. Food is Medicine

I read numerous books, journals, and research papers. I discovered that some meals might aggravate inflammation while others can reduce it. Gluten, dairy, and processed sweets are out. Nutrient-dense vegetables, lean meats, and healthy fats are in. My kitchen transformed into a sanctuary, a place where I could wield healing power.

2. Elimination Phase

I said farewell to gluten as if it were a long-time friend. It wasn't easy—the cravings, the social occasions with plentiful bread—but I persisted. Slowly, the fog lifted. My energy levels increased, and my skin recovered its luster. I discovered the superheroes of my new diet: quinoa, sweet potatoes, and avocado.

3. The Recipe Revolution.

Cookbooks became my pals. I experimented with flavors, adjusted recipes, and discovered the joys of cauliflower rice and zoodles. My mornings began with green smoothies containing kale, spinach, and a dash of hope. Lunches featured colorful salads with grilled chicken or chickpeas. What about dinner? Oh, the joys of a coconut curry or fish fillet with roasted Brussels sprouts.

4. Mindful eating.

I learned how to listen to my body. Was it yearning for warmth? A cup of nutritious soup awaited. Was stress threatening to derail me? Herbal drinks and meditation came to my rescue. I enjoyed every meal, thankful for the therapeutic properties of each ingredient.

5. Community & Connection

On this adventure, I discovered my tribe. Online forums, support groups, and Instagram hashtags—people who understood the struggle, victories, and setbacks. We compared recipes, celebrated achievements, and encouraged each other. Hashimoto's was no longer a one-on-one battle; it was a team effort to achieve wellness.

The Transformation

Months passed into years. The scale no longer determined my worth. Instead, I evaluated success in terms of energy, mental clarity, and the lack of joint pain. My thyroid antibodies dropped, and my heart overflowed with gratitude. Hashimoto's diet was more than simply food; it was about reclaiming my life.

A New Chapter.

So, as I finish this intro, I will welcome you to the recipes in these pages. Let them serve you as compass and armor against the storm. May they nourish you not just physically, but also spiritually. We find healing in the kitchen and strength in our stories.

Remember: you are not alone. We rise together, one good meal at a time.

With love and resilience.

Your fellow Hashimoto's warrior.

Understanding Hashimoto's Thyroiditis

Hashimoto's thyroiditis is an autoimmune condition in which the body's defense system attacks its tissues. In this situation, the immune system targets the thyroid gland, a small, butterfly-shaped organ near the base of the neck. This gland regulates your body's metabolism by generating hormones that control energy consumption.

When you have Hashimoto's, your immune system produces antibodies that target the thyroid as it is a foreign intruder. Over time, this assault might cause thyroid cells to become incapable of producing enough hormones, resulting in hypothyroidism.

Hashimoto's symptoms can be modest and build over time. You may feel especially weary, notice your skin growing dry, or discover that your hair is thinning. Some persons develop weight gain, muscle pains, and sensitivity to cold. It's as if your internal temperature and energy regulator are out of rhythm, making you feel off-balance.

Hashimoto's is commonly diagnosed through blood tests that check for thyroid antibodies and evaluate hormone levels. Synthetic hormones are frequently used as part of treatment to replace what your thyroid can no longer produce.

It is a condition that requires collaboration with your healthcare practitioner to manage and monitor, but with the appropriate approach, you can live a healthy and active lifestyle. It's all about listening to your body, interpreting its cues, and responding with caution.

The importance of diet in managing Hashimoto's

The role of food in managing Hashimoto's Thyroiditis cannot be overemphasized. This autoimmune illness, in which the body's immune system erroneously assaults the thyroid gland, can cause a series of symptoms that impair a person's quality of life. The thyroid gland, which regulates metabolism, heart rate, and body temperature, becomes impaired, resulting in hypothyroidism. Hashimoto's symptoms are usually modest and include fatigue, weight gain, cold intolerance, and dry skin.

Diet is crucial in treating these symptoms and the disease's overall course. While medicine is essential for treatment, dietary choices can have a substantial impact on the inflammatory processes that cause Hashimoto's. Inflammation is a major factor in the development and progression of autoimmune diseases, and many foods can either increase or reduce inflammation.

Foods to embrace and avoid

Foods high in omega-3 fatty acids, such as fatty fish, flaxseeds, and walnuts, can help lower inflammation. Antioxidant-rich fruits and vegetables such as berries, spinach, and bell peppers boost the immune system and protect the thyroid gland from oxidative stress.

Conversely, certain foods might aggravate inflammation and should be avoided. Gluten, which is contained in wheat, barley, and rye, has been related to increased intestinal permeability and may cause an immunological response in sensitive individuals. Similarly, some Hashimoto patients may have difficulty eating dairy products due to lactose intolerance or casein sensitivity.

Supplements and Nutrients

Nutritional supplements can also help manage Hashimoto's. Selenium and zinc are necessary for thyroid function and can be found in foods such as Brazil nuts, pumpkin seeds, and oysters. Vitamin D, which is typically inadequate in people with autoimmune illnesses, is essential for immune modulation and can be gained by sun exposure and fortified foods.

Lifestyle Modifications

Beyond diet, lifestyle factors like stress management and exercise are critical. Chronic stress can exacerbate autoimmune responses, therefore relaxation practices such as meditation, yoga, and deep breathing exercises are beneficial. Regular physical activity can aid with weight management, mood improvement, and stress reduction, all of which are beneficial to persons with Hashimoto's.

Individualized Approach.

It's crucial to remember that there is no one-size-fits-all diet for Hashimoto's. Each person reacts differently to different foods, so what works for one person may not work for another. An elimination diet, in which potentially troublesome foods are removed and then progressively reintroduced, can aid in identifying personal triggers.

The Role of Healthcare Professionals

Working with a healthcare practitioner or dietician can help you make nutritional modifications based on your specific needs and preferences. They can assist in the development of a personalized food plan that targets specific symptoms while also supporting general thyroid health.

Conclusion

Finally, food is an effective aid for managing Hashimoto's thyroiditis. Individuals can control their symptoms and enhance their quality of life by eating anti-inflammatory foods, avoiding potential triggers, and supplementing with important nutrients. Dietary management, when combined with lifestyle changes and medical treatment, is the foundation of a comprehensive approach to living with Hashimoto's.

How Can This Cookbook Help

This cookbook, created exclusively for those dealing with the problems of Hashimoto's Hypothyroidism, is more than just a collection of dishes; it's a guide on your path to wellness. Here's how it can assist.

Empowerment Through Education: It begins with demystifying Hashimoto's disease, explaining how nutrition affects your illness, and providing you with the knowledge you need to make informed food choices.

Personalized Nutrition: By focusing on anti-inflammatory foods and eliminating common triggers such as gluten and dairy, the recipes are designed to lower thyroid stress, potentially alleviating symptoms and regulating hormone levels.

Symptom Management: By delivering meals tailored to the specific needs of Hashimoto's patients, this cookbook can help control common symptoms including fatigue, weight gain, and brain fog, thereby improving your overall quality of life.

Emotional Support: The cookbook recognizes the emotional aspects of living with an autoimmune disease, providing comfort via nutritional meals that do not feel like a sacrifice, thereby supporting both your physical and emotional well-being.

Community Connection: It connects you to people who share your experiences, providing you with a sense of belonging and understanding that can be therapeutic in and of itself.

Lifestyle Integration: In addition to recipes, the cookbook provides advice on meal planning, preparation, and lifestyle changes that may be incorporated into your treatment plan, making Hashimoto's management a seamless part of your life.

In essence, this cookbook is a handbook that acknowledges the complexities of Hashimoto's disease and offers practical, everyday solutions for living a healthier, more balanced lifestyle. It demonstrates that, with the appropriate approach, eating can be both medicinal a

Chapter 1: The Hashimoto's Healing Diet

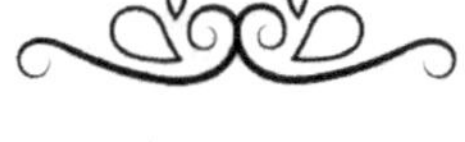

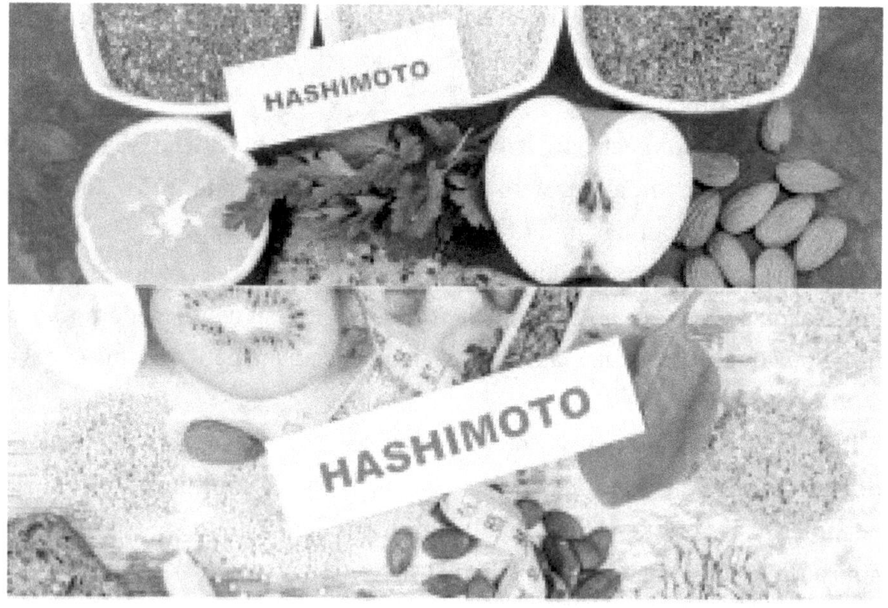

Key Dietary Principles for Hashimoto's

Dietary management of Hashimoto's Hypothyroidism requires a grasp of the complex link between food and the autoimmune response. The primary dietary principles for Hashimoto's are to reduce inflammation, support thyroid function, and balance hormones. Here's a full analysis of these principles:

1. Eat Anti-Inflammatory Foods: Inflammation is a major factor in Hashimoto's progression. An anti-inflammatory diet consists of foods high in omega-3 fatty acids, antioxidants, and phytonutrients. Fatty fish such as salmon, flaxseeds, chia seeds, and walnuts are high in omega-3s. Colorful fruits and vegetables, such as berries, leafy greens, and cruciferous vegetables like broccoli and cauliflower, contain antioxidants that help fight oxidative stress.

2. Eliminate Gluten and Grains: A gluten-free or grain-free diet can help alleviate symptoms of Hashimoto's disease. Gluten, a protein present in wheat, barley, and rye, can elicit an immunological response and worsen thyroid problems. Grains, in general, can lead to inflammation and should be limited or avoided.

3. Avoid Dairy Products: Hashimoto's patients may have lactose intolerance or sensitivity to casein, a protein found in dairy. Eliminating dairy from your diet may help reduce inflammation and improve digestion.

4. Focus on Nutrient Density:

A diet high in nutrient-dense, whole foods has the vitamins and minerals required for thyroid function. Selenium and zinc, present in Brazil nuts and pumpkin seeds help thyroid hormone production. Seaweed and fish are good sources of iodine, which is important for thyroid function. However, iodine intake should be controlled because too much might be harmful.

5. Limit intake of goitrogens, which can disrupt thyroid function. They are found in foods such as soy, peanuts, and cruciferous vegetables. Cooking these meals can lessen their goitrogenic properties.

6. Maintain a Balanced Fiber Intake: Fiber is essential for digestive health, which is typically affected in Hashimoto's patients. A diet rich in fiber from vegetables, fruits, and legumes can improve intestinal health and regularity.

7. Maintaining stable blood sugar levels is essential for managing

Hashimoto's. A diet low in refined carbohydrates and sugars, but high in fiber and healthy fats, can help minimize blood sugar surges that can cause inflammation.

8. Stay Hydrated: Staying hydrated is crucial for good health and helps alleviate Hashimoto's symptoms. Water aids in the elimination of pollutants and the regulation of metabolic processes.

9. Avoid processed foods with additives, preservatives, and unhealthy fats, which can cause inflammation. A whole-food diet reduces exposure to these possible irritants.

10. Practice Mindful Eating: Be present and attentive to the eating experience. It improves comprehension of hunger cues, enhances digestion, and can lead to more intelligent eating choices.

11. Use supplements wisely: Vitamin D, B vitamins, and probiotics help improve thyroid and immunological function. However, supplementation should be done with the supervision of a healthcare expert.

12. Personalize Your Diet: Hashimoto's patients may have unique dietary requirements and sensitivities. A personalized strategy, which may include an elimination diet, might help you determine what works best for you.

13. Collaborate with Healthcare Professionals: Working with a dietitian or nutritionist who understands Hashimoto's can assist design a food plan to your specific needs, ensuring you get the nutrients you need without increasing symptoms.

14. Regular Monitoring and Adjustment: As your condition changes, so may your nutritional requirements. Regular check-ins with your healthcare practitioner might help you alter your diet to match your changing needs.

In conclusion, the essential dietary principles for Hashimoto's disease include a focus on anti-inflammatory foods, removal of possible triggers such as gluten and dairy, and a tailored approach to nutrition. Individuals suffering from Hashimoto's disease can enhance their overall well-being by following these ideas.

Preparing Your Hashimoto's-Friendly Kitchen

Setting up a Hashimoto 's-friendly kitchen is a game-changing move toward better health and well-being. It's about making an environment that accommodates your dietary demands and makes it easier to prepare meals that fuel your body while also soothing your thyroid. Here's how to design a kitchen atmosphere that supports your health goals:

1. Clear the Space: Start by organizing your kitchen. Remove foods that are not good for your Hashimoto's diet, such as gluten, dairy, soy, and high sugars. This helps to reduce cross-contamination and temptation.

2. Stock your pantry with Hashimoto 's-friendly products. Gluten-free grains such as quinoa and brown rice, legumes, nuts, seeds, and coconut aminos, can be used as a substitute for soy sauce. Cook with healthy oils such as olive oil and avocado oil.

3. Create a fresh produce section in your refrigerator. These should form the foundation of your diet, supplying critical vitamins, minerals, and antioxidants.

4. Organize for Convenience: Arrange kitchen tools and supplies for easy meal prep. Keep commonly used things within easy reach, and group comparable items, such as baking ingredients or spices.

5. Purchase high-quality cookware, including non-stick pans, knives, and glass storage containers, for safer and more enjoyable food preparation.

6. Create a Herb and Spice Haven: Adding herbs and spices to your dishes not only enhances flavor but also provides health advantages. Create a separate area for turmeric, ginger, cinnamon, and other thyroid-supporting spices.

7. Choose Safe Cookware: Select cookware free of heavy metals and hazardous chemicals. Ceramic, cast iron and stainless steel are all wonderful choices that do not leach harmful elements into your food.

8. Use kitchen equipment like slow cookers, blenders, and food processors to prepare Hashimoto's-friendly foods and stick to your diet.

9. Set aside time each week for food prep. Prepare veggies, cereals, and

proteins in advance. This will save you time while also ensuring that you always have healthy options available.

10. Keep your kitchen clean to minimize mold and bacteria growth, which can impair a vulnerable immune system.

11. Label all containers with their contents and expiration dates. This helps you keep track of your food and minimizes waste.

12. Create a Recipe Collection: Collect your favorite Hashimoto's-friendly dishes. Keep them in a binder or digital format for convenient reference while planning meals.

13. Educate Household Members: If you live with others, inform them about your dietary needs and the necessity of maintaining a Hashimoto-friendly kitchen.

14. Plan Your Shopping: Create a grocery list based on your weekly meal plan. Stick to the periphery of the supermarket, where fresh produce, meats, and other whole items are usually found.

15. Avoid Cross-Contamination: If you share a kitchen with non-Hashimoto's dieters, be mindful of cross-contamination risks. Use different cutting boards and tools for gluten-free and gluten-containing dishes.

16. Embrace Fermentation: Incorporate fermented foods into your diet for probiotic advantages. You may set up a tiny fermenting station in your kitchen to make homemade sauerkraut or kombucha.

17. Prioritize Hydration: Use a decent water filter to remove pollutants from your drinking water. Staying hydrated is critical to overall wellness.

18. Be flexible with your kitchen setup as your demands may alter over time. This could be exploring new cuisine or replacing tools that no longer serve you.

19. Find Inspiration: Inspire yourself by following Hashimoto 's-friendly food bloggers, participating in online networks, or reading thyroid-related magazines.

20. Recognize Your Hard Work: Celebrate your efforts in controlling your health. Each step you take to create a Hashimoto's-friendly kitchen is one step closer to a healthier you.

By changing your kitchen into a health haven, you gain control over your Hashimoto's management. It's not just about what you eat; it's also about developing a lifestyle that supports your path to well-being. With each meal cooked in your Hashimoto 's-friendly kitchen, you fuel your body while also honoring your health. Remember that the path to health is about creating a caring atmosphere along the way, not just arriving at your destination.

Chapter 2: The 3-Day Kickstart Cleanse

Purpose and Benefits of Cleanse

A nutritional cleansing serves multiple purposes in the treatment of Hashimoto's hypothyroidism. It seeks to reset the body's systems, notably the digestive and immunological systems, which are frequently damaged in autoimmune disorders such as Hashimoto's. The benefits of such a cleanse are numerous, and it can result in a considerable increase in general health.

Purpose of the cleanse:

1. Reduce Inflammation: The cleanse's primary purpose is to reduce systemic inflammation, which is a major contributor to autoimmune reactions. By removing potential dietary triggers, the cleanse can help to calm the immune system and reduce thyroid gland inflammation.

2. Eliminate Toxins: The cleanse is intended to enhance the body's natural detoxification processes by removing toxins that may contribute to the autoimmune response.

3. uncover Food Sensitivities: By eliminating particular foods and gradually returning them, the cleanse can help uncover specific food sensitivities that may exacerbate Hashimoto's symptoms.

4. Heal the Gut: A healthy gut is essential for a functioning immune system. The cleanse focuses on foods that promote gut health and may reduce intestinal permeability, often known as 'leaky gut,' which is frequently linked to autoimmune illnesses.

5. Support Thyroid Function: The cleanse contains minerals needed for thyroid health, such as selenium, zinc, and omega-3 fatty acids, which can help with thyroid hormone production and conversion.

6. Boost Energy Levels: By removing items that produce blood sugar spikes and crashes, the cleanse might assist in maintaining energy throughout the day.

7. Promote Weight Management: Weight gain is a common Hashimoto symptom caused by a sluggish metabolism. The cleanse can help you lose weight by focusing on full, unadulterated meals that promote metabolic health.

8. Improve Digestive Health: Digestive problems are typical in Hashimoto's. The cleanse seeks to enhance digestive function by using fiber-rich foods that encourage regularity and probiotics that help maintain healthy gut microbiota.

9. Improve Nutrient Absorption: By repairing the intestines and lowering inflammation, the cleanse can help the body absorb and use nutrients from food.

10. Develop Healthy Eating Habits: The cleanse lays the groundwork for long-term dietary adjustments that can maintain the health advantages and aid in the continuing management of Hashimoto's.

Benefits of the Cleanse

1. Symptom Relief: Many people experience a decrease in Hashimoto's symptoms, such as weariness, joint pain, and brain fog, after a cleanse.

2. Improved Immune Regulation: The cleanse may help balance the immune system, potentially decreasing the frequency and severity of autoimmune flare-ups.

3. Improved Hormone Balance: By boosting thyroid function and reducing

stress on the adrenal glands, the cleanse can help to achieve a more balanced hormonal profile.

4. Improved Mental Clarity: A processed-food-free, nutrient-dense diet can increase cognitive function and clarity.

5. Increased Vitality: Because the cleanse focuses on nutrient-dense foods, you may feel more energized and well-balanced overall.

6. Healthier Skin: The skin frequently reflects inside wellness. A cleansing that decreases inflammation can result in clearer, more vibrant skin.

7. Stabilized Mood: The link between nutrition and mood is widely understood. The cleanse can help to moderate mood fluctuations by giving a consistent supply of nutrients and preventing sugar highs and lows.

8. Long-Term Health Benefits: By encouraging a healthy lifestyle, the cleanse may reduce the likelihood of developing additional Hashimoto-related health conditions, such as cardiovascular disease and diabetes.

9. Empowerment Over Health: Participating in a cleanse can give you a sense of control and empowerment over your health, which is especially essential for people who have chronic diseases.

10. Community and Support: Cleanses are frequently conducted in groups or with the assistance of a healthcare provider, which fosters a sense of community and accountability.

Daily Meal Plans and Recipes

Day 1:
   - Breakfast: Avocado and Spinach Smoothie.
   - Lunch: Quinoa salad with roasted vegetables.
   - Dinner: baked salmon with steamed broccoli and sweet potatoes.
   Day 2:
   -Breakfast: Chia Pudding with Fresh Berries.
   - Lunch: lentil soup with kale.
   - Dinner: Grilled chicken breast with asparagus and brown rice.
   Day 3:

- Breakfast: Gluten-free oatmeal with apple slices and cinnamon.
- Lunch: Turkey lettuce wraps with avocado.
Dinner: Beef Stir-Fry with Mixed Bell Peppers and Cauliflower Rice.
Day 4:
-Breakfast: Berry and Banana Protein Smoothie.
- Lunch: Spinach and mixed greens salad with grilled shrimp.
- Dinner: Roasted pork loin, green beans, and mashed butternut squash.
Day 5:
-Breakfast: Scrambled eggs with sautéed spinach and mushrooms.
Lunch: Chicken and Vegetable Soup
- Dinner: Baked cod with zucchini noodles and cherry tomatoes.
Day 6:
-Breakfast: Coconut yogurt with flax seeds and kiwi.
- Lunch: Chickpea salad with cucumbers and tomatoes.
- Dinner: Lamb chops with roasted Brussels sprouts and quinoa.
Day 7:
-Breakfast: Green juice with celery, cucumber, and ginger.
- Lunch: Sardine salad with mixed leafy greens.
Dinner: Stuffed bell peppers with ground turkey and vegetables.
Day 8:
-Breakfast: Pumpkin Seed and Almond Granola with Almond Milk.
- Lunch: Tuna Salad, Stuffed Avocado
Dinner: Lemon Garlic Shrimp with Steamed Broccoli and Wild Rice.
Day 9:
-Breakfast: Smoothie bowl with spinach, avocado, and chia seeds.
- Lunch: Roasted beet and carrot salad with walnuts.
- Dinner: Grilled tilapia with mixed vegetables and millet.
Day 10:
-Breakfast: Poached eggs with sautéed greens.
- Lunch: Butternut squash soup.
Dinner: Turkey Meatballs with Tomato Sauce and Spaghetti Squash.

Each meal is meant to give a balanced intake of protein, healthy fats, and carbohydrates, as well as foods high in selenium, zinc, and antioxidants. The dishes would be simple to prepare, made with nutritious foods, and free of frequent Hashimoto's triggers. It's crucial to note that individual nutritional demands differ, therefore changes may be required depending on health and preferences. Instructions and methods of cooking are explained later in the book.

Tips for a Successful Cleanse

When you have Hashimoto's Hypothyroidism, doing a food cleanse can be a significant step toward better health. Here are specific suggestions for a successful cleanse:

1. Seek advice from a healthcare professional before beginning a cleanse, especially if you have an autoimmune disorder like Hashimoto's. They can offer advice targeted to your specific health requirements.
2. Avoid foods that cause Hashimoto's symptoms, including gluten, dairy, soy, and processed carbohydrates. These can cause inflammation and worsen thyroid disorders.
3. Incorporate Anti-Inflammatory Foods into Your Diet. Omega-3-rich foods include fatty fish, berries, almonds, and leafy greens.
4. Stay Hydrated: Drink plenty of water during the cleanse. Proper water can help remove toxins from your system and improve your overall health.
5. Promote Gut Health: Incorporate probiotic-rich foods, such as fermented vegetables, or take a high-quality probiotic supplement, to maintain a healthy gut flora, which is crucial for immune function.
6. Prioritize Sleep: Ensure you receive enough sleep during the cleanse. Sleep is crucial for your body's healing and rejuvenation.
7. Reduce Stress: Practice stress-reduction techniques like meditation, yoga, or deep breathing exercises. Chronic stress can weaken the immune system and impede the cleansing process.

8. Engage in light exercise, such as walking or swimming. Physical activity can improve circulation and detoxification without overworking the body.

9. Nutrient-Dense Whole Foods: Eat whole foods to get key nutrients without extra preservatives and chemicals from processed foods.

10. Limit consumption of goitrogenic foods, such as raw cruciferous vegetables, as these can disrupt thyroid function. Cooking these meals can lessen their goitrogenic properties.

11. Include Selenium and Zinc: These minerals are essential for thyroid function. Foods rich in selenium and zinc include Brazil nuts, pumpkin seeds, and oysters.

12. Gradual Reintroduction: After cleansing, gently reintroduce meals to monitor your body's reaction and discover any dietary sensitivities.

13. Pay attention to your body's responses during the detox. If you suffer any side effects, speak with your doctor.

14. Keep a journal to document your experience, including food intake, mood, and symptom changes. This can assist uncover trends and inform future dietary decisions.

15. Plan: Prepare meals ahead of time to prevent choosing unhealthy options.

16. Seek Support: Join a community or join a support group for those managing Hashimoto's. Sharing experiences and tips can be beneficial.

17. Consume high-quality proteins such as organic chicken, grass-fed beef, and wild-caught fish to maintain muscle strength and metabolism during the cleanse.

18. Consume healthy fats like avocados, olive oil, and coconut oil to promote hormone balance and energy.

19. Avoid Harsh Detoxes: Avoid harsh detox techniques that offer speedy results. These can be harsh on your body and may not be suitable for people who have Hashimoto's.

20. Continuous Learning: Remain knowledgeable about Hashimoto's and how diet affects your health. Research is ongoing, and fresh discoveries can help you improve your health-management strategy.

A successful Hashimoto's cleanse is about more than simply the things you eat; it's about creating a healthy environment for your body to heal and thrive in. Remember that the purpose is to nourish and restore your body, not to deny it. Following these guidelines will ensure that your cleanse is not only successful but also a great beginning toward long-term health management.

Chapter 3: Breakfast

Smoothies and Juices

Here is a smoothie and juice recipes tailored for Hashimoto's Thyroiditis, focusing on anti-inflammatory ingredients and thyroid-supporting nutrients:

1. **Berry Thyroid-Boost Smoothie**
   - Ingredients:
   - 1 cup mixed berries (strawberries, blueberries, raspberries)
   - 1 banana
   - 1 cup spinach
   - 1 tablespoon chia seeds
   - 1 cup unsweetened almond milk
   - 1 scoop protein powder (optional)

- Instructions:

   1. Combine all ingredients in a blender.
   2. Blend until smooth.
   3. Serve immediately.

- Time: 5 minutes

   - Nutritional Information: Rich in antioxidants, fiber, and omega-3 fatty acids.

2. Green Thyroid Warrior Juice

   - Ingredients:
   - 2 cups kale or spinach
   - 1 green apple
   - 1/2 cucumber
   - 1/2 lemon, juiced
   - 1 inch ginger root

- Instructions

   1. Wash all produce thoroughly.
   2. Juice all ingredients in a juicer.
   3. Stir in lemon juice and enjoy.

- Time: 10 minutes

   - Nutritional Information: High in vitamins A, C, and K, and anti-inflammatory properties.

3. Selenium Power Smoothie

   - Ingredients:
   - 2 Brazil nuts (rich in selenium)
   - 1 cup spinach
   - 1/2 avocado
   - 1 cup coconut water
   - 1/2 cup pineapple chunks

- Instructions:

   1. Blend Brazil nuts and spinach with coconut water until smooth.

2. Add avocado and pineapple; blend again.
3. Serve chilled.

- Time: 5 minutes
    - Nutritional Information: Excellent source of selenium and healthy fats.

4. **Anti-inflammatory turmeric Smoothie**
    - Ingredients:
    - 1 cup coconut milk
    - 1/2 teaspoon turmeric powder
    - 1/2 teaspoon cinnamon
    - 1 banana
    - 1 tablespoon almond butter
    - 1 teaspoon honey (optional)

- Instructions:

    1. Combine all ingredients in a blender.
    2. Blend until creamy.
    3. Serve immediately.

- Time: 5 minutes
    - Nutritional Information: Contains anti-inflammatory turmeric and heart-healthy fats.

5. **Gut-Healing Probiotic Juice**
    - Ingredients:
    - 1/2 cup sauerkraut juice
    - 1 cup carrot juice
    - 1/2 apple
    - 1/2 lemon, juiced

- Instructions:

1. Combine sauerkraut juice, carrot juice, and apple in a blender.
2. Blend until smooth.
3. Stir in lemon juice and serve.

- Time: 5 minutes
   - Nutritional Information: Probiotic-rich with digestive benefits.

6. **Thyroid-Supporting Berry Juice**
   - Ingredients:
   - 1 cup strawberries
   - 1/2 cup cranberries
   - 1/2 cup blackberries
   - 1/2 cup water or coconut water

- Instructions:

1. Blend all berries with water until smooth.
2. Strain through a fine mesh if desired.
3. Serve chilled.

- Time: 5 minutes
   - Nutritional Information: Packed with vitamin C and antioxidants.

7. **Detox Green Juice**
   - Ingredients:
   - 2 cups mixed greens (spinach, kale, chard)
   - 1/2 cucumber
   - 2 celery stalks
   - 1/2 green apple
   - 1/2 lemon, juiced

- Instructions:

1. Juice all ingredients except lemon in a juicer.
2. Stir in lemon juice and drink immediately.

- Time: 10 minutes
    - Nutritional Information: Detoxifying and rich in chlorophyll.

8. **Omega-3 Rich Flaxseed Smoothie**
    - Ingredients:
    - 1 tablespoon ground flaxseed
    - 1 cup unsweetened almond milk
    - 1 banana
    - 1/2 cup frozen mango chunks
    - 1/2 teaspoon vanilla extract

- Instructions:

1. Blend all ingredients until smooth.
2. Serve immediately.

- Time: 5 minutes
    - Nutritional Information: High in omega-3 fatty acids and fiber.

9. **Refreshing Cucumber Mint Juice**
    - Ingredients:
    - 1 large cucumber
    - A handful of fresh mint leaves
    - 1/2 lime, juiced
    - 1/2 cup water

- Instructions:

1. Juice cucumber and mint leaves.
2. Stir in lime juice and water.

3. Serve over ice.

- Time: 5 minutes
  - Nutritional Information: Hydrating and refreshing with digestive benefits.

10. **Zinc Booster Smoothie**
    - Ingredients:
    - 1/2 cup pumpkin seeds (rich in zinc)
    - 1 cup unsweetened almond milk
    - 1 banana
    - 1/2 cup frozen blueberries
    - 1 scoop protein powder (optional)

- Instructions:

  1. Blend pumpkin seeds and almond milk until smooth.
  2. Add the remaining ingredients and blend again.
  3. Serve chilled.

- Time: 5 minutes
  - Nutritional Information: Excellent source of zinc and antioxidants.
  These recipes are designed to be nutrient-dense, focusing on ingredients that support thyroid health and reduce inflammation.

Gluten-Free Pancakes and Waffles

Gluten-free pancake and waffle recipes suitable for managing Hashimoto's Thyroiditis, focusing on ingredients that support thyroid health and avoid common dietary triggers:

1. **Basic Gluten-Free Pancakes**
   - Ingredients:
   - 1 cup gluten-free all-purpose flour

  - 1 tablespoon sugar
  - 2 teaspoons baking powder
  - 1/2 teaspoon salt
  - 1 cup almond milk
  - 2 tablespoons vegetable oil
  - 1 egg

- Instructions:

  1. Mix the dry ingredients.
  2. In another bowl, whisk the wet ingredients.
  3. Combine both mixtures until smooth.
  4. Cook on a hot griddle until golden brown.

- Time: 20 minutes
  - Nutritional Information: Approximately 150 calories per pancake, with essential nutrients from the gluten-free flour blend.

2. Almond Flour Waffles
  - Ingredients:
  - 2 cups almond flour
  - 1 teaspoon baking soda
  - 1/4 teaspoon salt
  - 2 eggs
  - 1/2 cup water
  - 1/3 cup coconut oil, melted
  - 1 tablespoon maple syrup

- Instructions:

  1. Combine dry ingredients in a bowl.
  2. Mix wet ingredients in another bowl.
  3. Blend both until smooth.

4. Pour into a heated waffle iron and cook until crispy.

- Time: 15 minutes

   - Nutritional Information: Rich in protein and healthy fats, around 300 calories per waffle.

3. Coconut Flour Pancakes
   - Ingredients:
   - 1/4 cup coconut flour
   - 1/8 teaspoon baking soda
   - Pinch of salt
   - 1/4 cup coconut milk
   - 2 eggs
   - 1 tablespoon honey
   - 1/2 teaspoon vanilla extract

- Instructions:

   1. Sift together the dry ingredients.
   2. Whisk the wet ingredients in a separate bowl.
   3. Combine and mix until there are no lumps.
   4. Cook on a skillet over medium heat.

- Time: 25 minutes

   - Nutritional Information: Low carb, high fiber, about 100 calories per pancake.

4. Banana Oat Waffles
   - Ingredients:
   - 2 ripe bananas, mashed
   - 1 1/2 cups gluten-free oats
   - 1 cup almond milk
   - 2 eggs

  - 1 teaspoon vanilla extract
  - 1 teaspoon cinnamon

- Instructions:

  1. Blend oats to make flour.
  2. Mix all ingredients until smooth.
  3. Cook in a waffle iron until browned.

- Time: 20 minutes
  - Nutritional Information: Nutrient-dense, approximately 280 calories per waffle.

5. **Apple Cinnamon Pancakes**
  - Ingredients:
  - 1 cup gluten-free all-purpose flour
  - 1 apple, grated
  - 1 teaspoon cinnamon
  - 1 teaspoon baking powder
  - 1/4 teaspoon salt
  - 1 cup almond milk
  - 1 egg
  - 1 tablespoon coconut oil

- Instructions:

  1. Mix flour, cinnamon, baking powder, and salt.
  2. Combine milk, egg, and oil in another bowl.
  3. Stir in the grated apple.
  4. Cook on a griddle until each side is golden.

- Time: 30 minutes
  - Nutritional Information: A good source of fiber, around 160 calories per

pancake.

6. **Pumpkin Spice Waffles**

   - Ingredients:
   - 2 cups gluten-free all-purpose flour
   - 1/4 cup brown sugar
   - 1 tablespoon baking powder
   - 2 teaspoons pumpkin spice
   - 1/2 teaspoon salt
   - 1 1/2 cups almond milk
   - 1 cup pumpkin puree
   - 1 egg
   - 2 tablespoons coconut oil

- Instructions:

   1. Whisk together dry ingredients.
   2. In a separate bowl, mix wet ingredients.
   3. Combine and stir until smooth.
   4. Pour batter into a preheated waffle iron.

- Time: 25 minutes
   - Nutritional Information: High in vitamin A, about 260 calories per waffle.

7. **Blueberry Lemon Pancakes**

   - Ingredients:
   - 1 cup gluten-free all-purpose flour
   - 1 teaspoon baking powder
   - 1/4 teaspoon salt
   - Zest of 1 lemon
   - 1 cup almond milk
   - 1 egg
   - 1 tablespoon coconut oil

- 1/2 cup fresh blueberries

- Instructions:

  1. Combine flour, baking powder, salt, and lemon zest.
  2. Mix in milk, egg, and oil until smooth.
  3. Gently fold in blueberries.
  4. Cook on a hot griddle, flipping once.

- Time: 20 minutes
  - Nutritional Information: Rich in antioxidants, around 140 calories per pancake.

8. **Sweet Potato Waffles**
   - Ingredients:
   - 1 cup mashed sweet potato
   - 1 1/2 cups gluten-free all-purpose flour
   - 2 teaspoons baking powder
   - 1/2 teaspoon cinnamon
   - 1/4 teaspoon nutmeg
   - 1/4 teaspoon salt
   - 1 1/4 cups almond milk
   - 2 eggs
   - 1 tablespoon maple syrup

- Instructions:

  1. Mix flour, baking powder, spices, and salt.
  2. Whisk together sweet potato, milk, eggs, and syrup.
  3. Combine wet and dry ingredients.
  4. Cook in a waffle iron until crisp.

- Time: 30 minutes

- Nutritional Information: Good source of beta-carotene, about 250 calories per waffle.

9. Fluffy Rice Flour Pancakes

  - Ingredients:
  - 1 cup rice flour
  - 1 tablespoon sugar
  - 2 teaspoons baking powder
  - 1/2 teaspoon salt
  - 1 cup almond milk
  - 2 tablespoons vegetable oil
  - 1 egg

- Instructions:

  1. Mix dry ingredients in a bowl.
  2. In another bowl, whisk wet ingredients.
  3. Stir together until just combined.
  4. Pour batter onto a hot griddle and cook.

- Time: 20 minutes
  - Nutritional Information: Light and easy to digest, around 130 calories per pancake.

10. Chocolate Chip Buckwheat Waffles

  - Ingredients:
  - 1 1/2 cups buckwheat flour
  - 1/4 cup cocoa powder
  - 2 teaspoons baking powder
  - 1/4 teaspoon salt
  - 1 3/4 cups almond milk
  - 2 eggs
  - 1/4 cup melted coconut oil

- 1/3 cup chocolate chips

- Instructions:

1. Whisk together dry ingredients.
2. Mix in wet ingredients until smooth.
3. Fold in chocolate chips.
4. Cook in a waffle iron until done.

- Time: 25 minutes
- Nutritional Information: Rich in fiber and chocolatey goodness, approximately 320 calories per waffle.

These recipes provide a variety of flavors and nutrients suitable for a Hashimoto diet, ensuring you can enjoy a delicious breakfast without worrying about gluten or other common triggers.

Savory Breakfast Bowls

Savory breakfast bowls can be a nourishing and satisfying way to start the day, especially for managing Hashimoto's Hypothyroidism. Here are some ideas for savory breakfast bowls, complete with ingredients, instructions, and nutritional highlights:

1. **Quinoa and Veggie Bowl**
   - Ingredients:
   - 1/2 cup cooked quinoa
   - 1/4 cup sautéed spinach
   - 1/4 cup roasted cherry tomatoes
   - 1 soft-boiled egg
   - 1 tablespoon pumpkin seeds
   - Salt and pepper to taste

- Instructions:

1. Prepare quinoa according to package instructions.
2. Sauté spinach and roast cherry tomatoes.
3. Soft boil an egg.
4. Assemble all ingredients in a bowl.
5. Top with pumpkin seeds, salt, and pepper.

- Time: 20 minutes
- Nutritional Information: High in protein, fiber, and essential minerals like magnesium and zinc.

2. Turmeric Tofu Scramble
- Ingredients:
- 1/2 block firm tofu, crumbled
- 1/2 teaspoon turmeric
- 1/4 teaspoon garlic powder
- 1/4 cup diced bell peppers
- 1/4 cup diced onions
- 1 tablespoon olive oil
- Salt and pepper to taste

- Instructions:

1. Heat olive oil in a pan.
2. Sauté onions and bell peppers until soft.
3. Add crumbled tofu and turmeric, and cook for 5 minutes.
4. Season with garlic powder, salt, and pepper.
5. Serve warm.

- Time: 15 minutes
- Nutritional Information: Rich in plant-based protein and anti-inflammatory properties from turmeric.

3. **Sweet Potato Hash**
   - Ingredients:
   - 1 medium sweet potato, diced
   - 1/4 cup diced onion
   - 1/4 cup diced bell pepper
   - 2 tablespoons olive oil
   - 1/2 teaspoon smoked paprika
   - Salt and pepper to taste

- Instructions:

   1. Preheat the oven to 400°F (200°C).
   2. Toss sweet potatoes, onions, and bell peppers with olive oil, paprika, salt, and pepper.
   3. Spread on a baking sheet and roast until tender, about 20 minutes.
   4. Serve hot.

- Time: 30 minutes
   - Nutritional Information: Good source of complex carbohydrates and vitamin A.

4. **Avocado and Salmon Bowl**
   - Ingredients:
   - 1/2 avocado, sliced
   - 3 ounces smoked salmon
   - 1/4 cup cucumber, sliced
   - 1 tablespoon capers
   - 1/2 lemon, juiced
   - Salt and pepper to taste

- Instructions:

   1. Arrange avocado and smoked salmon in a bowl.

2. Add sliced cucumber and capers.
3. Drizzle with lemon juice.
4. Season with salt and pepper.

- Time: 10 minutes

   - Nutritional Information: High in omega-3 fatty acids and healthy monounsaturated fats.

5. **Kale and Mushroom Sauté**
   - Ingredients:
   - 1 cup kale, chopped
   - 1/2 cup mushrooms, sliced
   - 1 garlic clove, minced
   - 1 tablespoon olive oil
   - Salt and pepper to taste

- Instructions:

   1. Heat olive oil in a pan over medium heat.
   2. Add garlic and mushrooms, and sauté until browned.
   3. Add kale and cook until wilted.
   4. Season with salt and pepper.
   5. Serve warm.

- Time: 15 minutes

   - Nutritional Information: Rich in vitamins C and K, and a good source of iron and calcium.

These savory breakfast bowls are designed to be nutrient-dense, providing a balanced meal to support thyroid health. They avoid common Hashimoto's triggers like gluten and dairy and focus on anti-inflammatory and nutrient-rich ingredients.

Chapter 4: Lunch

Salads Full of Super foods

Salad recipes that are suitable for a Hashimoto's diet, focusing on ingredients that support thyroid health and avoid common triggers:

1. **Quinoa Fennel Salad**

- Ingredients:
- 1 cup cooked quinoa
- 1/2 cup chopped fennel
- 1/2 cup halved grapes
- 1/4 cup slivered almonds
- A few sprigs of fresh thyme
- Drizzle of olive oil
- Splash of red wine vinegar

- Instructions:

1. Combine the cooked quinoa, chopped fennel, and halved grapes in a bowl.
2. Add the slivered almonds and fresh thyme.

3. Drizzle with olive oil and red wine vinegar to taste.
4. Toss everything together and serve.

- Time: 15 minutes

- Nutritional Information: Quinoa is a complete protein source and rich in fiber, while fennel aids digestion.

2. **Ultimate Chopped Salad**
   - Ingredients:
   - 2 cups mixed greens
   - 1/2 cup diced tomatoes
   - 1/2 cup cucumber, chopped
   - 1/4 cup red onion, finely chopped
   - 1/4 cup cooked chickpeas
   - 1/4 cup sunflower seeds
   - Dressing of choice (olive oil and lemon juice recommended)

- Instructions:

   1. Chop all vegetables and place them in a large bowl.
   2. Add the cooked chickpeas and sunflower seeds.
   3. Toss with your dressing of choice.
   4. Serve immediately.

- Time: 10 minutes

- Nutritional Information: This salad is full of fiber, vitamins, and minerals, with a good balance of carbohydrates, protein, and healthy fats.

3. **Thyroid-Friendly Broccoli Salad**
   - Ingredients:
   - 1 head of broccoli, chopped
   - 2 stalks of celery, chopped
   - 1/4 red onion, diced

- 2 tablespoons dried cranberries
- 1 hard-boiled egg, chopped
- Dressing of choice (a simple vinaigrette works well)

- Instructions:

1. Combine the chopped broccoli, celery, and red onion in a bowl.
2. Add the dried cranberries and chopped hard-boiled egg.
3. Toss with your preferred dressing.
4. Chill before serving.

- Time: 20 minutes
- Nutritional Information: Broccoli is a cruciferous vegetable that supports detoxification, and eggs provide a good source of selenium.

4. **Salmon Avocado Salad**
   - Ingredients:
   - 2 cups mixed greens
   - 1/2 avocado, sliced
   - 4 ounces of grilled salmon
   - 1/4 cup cherry tomatoes, halved
   - 1 tablespoon pumpkin seeds
   - Lemon vinaigrette dressing

- Instructions:

1. Place mixed greens in a bowl.
2. Top with sliced avocado, grilled salmon, and cherry tomatoes.
3. Sprinkle with pumpkin seeds.
4. Drizzle with lemon vinaigrette dressing.
5. Serve and enjoy.

- Time: 15 minutes

- Nutritional Information: Salmon is an excellent source of omega-3 fatty acids, and avocado provides healthy monounsaturated fats.

5. **Mediterranean Tuna Salad**
   - Ingredients:
   - 1 can of tuna, drained
   - 2 cups spinach leaves
   - 1/2 cup cherry tomatoes, halved
   - 1/4 cup sliced black olives
   - 1/4 cup diced cucumber
   - Feta cheese (optional)
   - Olive oil and lemon juice for dressing

- Instructions:

   1. Spread spinach leaves as a base in a bowl.
   2. Add the tuna, cherry tomatoes, black olives, and cucumber.
   3. Crumble feta cheese on top if using.
   4. Dress with olive oil and lemon juice.
   5. Toss gently and serve.

- Time: 10 minutes

   - Nutritional Information: Tuna is a good source of protein and essential nutrients like vitamin D and selenium.

These salads are designed to be nutrient-rich, easy to prepare, and suitable for managing Hashimoto's Hypothyroidism.

Hearty Soups and Stews

Soup and Stew recipes that are suitable for a Hashimoto's diet, focusing on ingredients that support thyroid health and avoid common triggers:

1. **Ginger Carrot Pear Soup**
   - Ingredients:
   - 2 tablespoons olive oil
   - 4 large carrots, peeled and chopped
   - 1 onion, chopped
   - 1 pear, peeled and chopped
   - 4 cups bone broth
   - 1 tablespoon grated ginger
   - Salt and pepper to taste

- Instructions:

   1. Heat oil in a soup pot over medium heat.
   2. Add carrots and onion, and cook until onions are translucent.
   3. Add pear and cook until softened.
   4. Pour in bone broth, bring to a boil, then simmer until carrots are tender.
   5. Add ginger, and blend until smooth.
   6. Season with salt and pepper, serve warm[1].

- Time: 35 minutes
   - Nutritional Information: Rich in vitamins A and C, and ginger has anti-inflammatory properties.

2. **Hearty Chicken and Vegetable Stew**
   - Ingredients:
   - 2 tablespoons olive oil
   - 1 lb chicken breast, cubed
   - 2 carrots, sliced

- 2 celery stalks, sliced
- 1 onion, diced
- 4 cups chicken broth
- 1 teaspoon thyme
- Salt and pepper to taste

- Instructions:

1. In a large pot, heat olive oil over medium heat.
2. Add chicken and cook until browned.
3. Add vegetables and sauté for a few minutes.
4. Pour in broth, add thyme, and bring to a boil.
5. Reduce heat and simmer until vegetables are tender.
6. Season with salt and pepper, serve hot.

- Time: 45 minutes
- Nutritional Information: High in protein and fiber, with immune-boosting properties.

3. **Mushroom and Thyme Soup**
   - Ingredients:
   - 1 tablespoon olive oil
   - 2 garlic cloves, minced
   - 1 lb mushrooms, sliced
   - 1 teaspoon dried thyme
   - 1 teaspoon dried parsley
   - 1 teaspoon dried rosemary
   - 2 tablespoons balsamic vinegar
   - 2 tablespoons gluten-free flour
   - 4 cups vegetable broth

- Instructions:

1. Cook garlic in oil until fragrant.
2. Add mushrooms and herbs, and cook for 5 minutes.
3. Pour in vinegar, and cook for 2 more minutes.
4. Sprinkle it with flour, and cook for 2 minutes.
5. Add broth, bring to a boil, then simmer[3].

- Time: 30 minutes

- Nutritional Information: Mushrooms are a good source of selenium, which is essential for thyroid function.

4. **Butternut Squash and Apple Soup**
   - Ingredients:
   - 1 tablespoon olive oil
   - 1 butternut squash, peeled and cubed
   - 1 apple, peeled and chopped
   - 1 onion, chopped
   - 4 cups vegetable broth
   - 1/2 teaspoon cinnamon
   - 1/4 teaspoon nutmeg
   - Salt and pepper to taste

- Instructions:

1. Heat oil in a large pot.
2. Add squash, apple, and onion, and cook until softened.
3. Pour in broth, add spices, and bring to a boil.
4. Simmer until squash is tender.
5. Blend until smooth, season with salt and pepper.

- Time: 40 minutes

- Nutritional Information: Squash is high in vitamin A, and apples add fiber.

5. **Lentil and Kale Stew**
   - Ingredients:
   - 1 tablespoon olive oil
   - 1 onion, diced
   - 2 garlic cloves, minced
   - 1 cup lentils, rinsed
   - 4 cups vegetable broth
   - 2 cups kale, chopped
   - 1 teaspoon cumin
   - Salt and pepper to taste

- Instructions:

1. In a pot, heat oil over medium heat.
2. Sauté onion and garlic until translucent.
3. Add lentils and broth, and bring to a boil.
4. Reduce heat, and add kale and cumin.
5. Simmer until lentils are tender.
6. Season with salt and pepper, serve warm.

- Time: 50 minutes
   - Nutritional Information: Lentils provide plant-based protein and iron, while kale is rich in antioxidants.

Wraps and Sandwiches with Gluten-Free Breads

Wrap and sandwich ideas that are gluten-free and suitable for managing Hashimoto's Thyroiditis:

1. **Grilled Chicken Lettuce Wrap**
   - Ingredients:
   - Grilled chicken breast, sliced

- Large lettuce leaves
- Sliced avocado
- Shredded carrots
- Cucumber sticks
- Hummus or tahini sauce

- Instructions:

1. Lay out lettuce leaves.
2. Spread a thin layer of hummus or tahini sauce.
3. Place chicken, avocado, carrots, and cucumber on top.
4. Roll the lettuce leaves to form wraps.

- Time: 15 minutes
    - Nutritional Information: High in protein, healthy fats, and fiber.

2. **Turkey and Spinach Gluten-Free Sandwich**
    - Ingredients:
    - 2 slices of gluten-free bread
    - Sliced turkey breast
    - Fresh spinach leaves
    - Sliced tomato
    - Mustard or gluten-free mayo

- Instructions:

1. Toast the gluten-free bread slices.
2. Spread mustard or mayo on one side of each slice.
3. Layer turkey, spinach, and tomato between the bread.
4. Cut in half and serve.

- Time: 10 minutes
    - Nutritional Information: Lean protein source with vitamins A and C

from spinach and tomato.

3. **Tuna Salad Collard Green Wrap**
   - Ingredients:
   - Collard green leaves, blanched
   - Canned tuna, drained
   - Diced celery
   - Diced red onion
   - Chopped parsley
   - Olive oil and lemon juice dressing

- Instructions:

   1. Mix tuna, celery, onion, and parsley in a bowl.
   2. Dress with olive oil and lemon juice.
   3. Place the mixture on collard green leaves.
   4. Roll up and slice in half.

- Time: 20 minutes
   - Nutritional Information: Rich in omega-3 fatty acids and iron.

4. **Roasted Vegetable Quinoa Wrap**
   - Ingredients:
   - Gluten-free tortillas
   - Cooked quinoa
   - Roasted red peppers, zucchini, and eggplant
   - Arugula or mixed greens
   - Balsamic vinaigrette

- Instructions:

   1. Warm the tortillas.
   2. Spread a layer of quinoa on each tortilla.

3. Add roasted vegetables and greens.
4. Drizzle with balsamic vinaigrette, and roll up the wraps.

- Time: 30 minutes (if vegetables are pre-roasted)
   - Nutritional Information: High in plant-based protein and antioxidants.

5. **Egg Salad Gluten-Free Sandwich**
   - Ingredients:
   - 2 slices of gluten-free bread
   - Hard-boiled eggs, chopped
   - Chopped celery
   - Chopped green onions
   - Gluten-free mayo
   - Lettuce leaves

- Instructions:

1. In a bowl, mix eggs, celery, green onions, and mayo.
2. Toast the bread slices.
3. Spread the egg salad on one slice of bread and top with lettuce.
4. Cover with the other slice, cut in half, and serve.

- Time: 15 minutes
   - Nutritional Information: Good source of protein and essential vitamins.

These recipes provide a variety of nutrients and flavors while adhering to a gluten-free diet, which is often recommended for Hashimoto's to help manage inflammation and immune response.

Chapter 5: Dinner

Comforting One-Pot Meals

1. **Hearty Vegetable Stew**
   - Ingredients:
   - 2 tbsp olive oil
   - 1 onion, diced
   - 2 cloves garlic, minced
   - 2 carrots, diced
   - 2 celery stalks, diced
   - 1 zucchini, diced
   - 1 cup green beans, trimmed
   - 1 can diced tomatoes
   - 4 cups vegetable broth
   - 1 tsp dried basil
   - Salt and pepper to taste

- Instructions:

   1. Heat olive oil in a large pot over medium heat.
   2. Add onion and garlic, sauté until translucent.

3. Add carrots, celery, zucchini, and green beans, and cook for 5 minutes.
4. Stir in diced tomatoes and vegetable broth.
5. Season with basil, salt, and pepper.
6. Bring to a boil, then simmer for 20 minutes.

- Time: 40 minutes

- Nutritional Information: Rich in fiber and vitamins from the variety of vegetables.

2. **Lemon Herb Chicken and Rice**
   - Ingredients:
   - 1 tbsp olive oil
   - 4 chicken thighs
   - 1 onion, chopped
   - 2 cups chicken broth
   - 1 cup rice
   - 1 lemon, juiced and zested
   - 1 tsp dried thyme
   - Salt and pepper to taste

- Instructions:

   1. In a pot, heat olive oil and brown chicken thighs on both sides.
   2. Remove chicken and sauté onion until soft.
   3. Add chicken broth, rice, lemon juice, and zest.
   4. Place the chicken back in the pot.
   5. Season with thyme, salt, and pepper.
   6. Cover and simmer until rice is cooked, about 20 minutes.

- Time: 45 minutes

- Nutritional Information: Provides protein from chicken and is infused with vitamin C from lemon.

3. **Beef and Sweet Potato Chili**
   - Ingredients:
   - 1 lb ground beef
   - 1 onion, diced
   - 2 sweet potatoes, peeled and cubed
   - 1 can diced tomatoes
   - 1 can black beans, drained and rinsed
   - 2 cups beef broth
   - 1 tbsp chili powder
   - 1 tsp cumin
   - Salt and pepper to taste

- Instructions:

   1. Brown ground beef in a pot.
   2. Add onion and cook until soft.
   3. Stir in sweet potatoes, diced tomatoes, black beans, and beef broth.
   4. Season with chili powder, cumin, salt, and pepper.
   5. Simmer until sweet potatoes are tender, about 30 minutes.

- Time: 45 minutes
   - Nutritional Information: High in protein and beta-carotene from sweet potatoes.

4. **Turmeric Coconut Chicken Soup**
   - Ingredients:
   - 1 tbsp coconut oil
   - 1 onion, chopped
   - 2 cloves garlic, minced
   - 1 tbsp grated ginger
   - 1 tsp turmeric
   - 4 cups chicken broth
   - 1 can of coconut milk

- 2 chicken breasts, shredded
- 2 cups spinach
- Salt and pepper to taste

- Instructions:

1. Heat coconut oil in a pot.
2. Sauté onion, garlic, and ginger until fragrant.
3. Add turmeric and stir for a minute.
4. Pour in chicken broth and coconut milk, and bring to a simmer.
5. Add shredded chicken and spinach.
6. Season with salt and pepper, simmer for 10 minutes.

- Time: 30 minutes
- Nutritional Information: Rich in anti-inflammatory properties from turmeric and healthy fats from coconut milk.

5. **Mushroom and Brown Rice Risotto**
   - Ingredients:
   - 1 tbsp olive oil
   - 1 lb mushrooms, sliced
   - 1 onion, diced
   - 2 cloves garlic, minced
   - 1 cup brown rice
   - 4 cups vegetable broth
   - 1 tsp dried thyme
   - Salt and pepper to taste

- Instructions:

1. In a pot, heat olive oil and sauté mushrooms until browned.
2. Add onion and garlic, and cook until soft.
3. Stir in brown rice until well coated.

4. Gradually add vegetable broth, stirring constantly.
5. Season with thyme, salt, and pepper.
6. Simmer until rice is tender and creamy, about 45 minutes.

- Time: 1 hour

   - Nutritional Information: Brown rice provides fiber and mushrooms are a good source of selenium.

Protein-Packed Main Courses

1. **Grilled Lemon-Garlic Salmon**
   - Ingredients:
   - 4 salmon filets
   - 2 lemons (1 juiced, 1 sliced)
   - 2 garlic cloves, minced
   - 2 tbsp olive oil
   - Fresh dill
   - Salt and pepper to taste

- Instructions:

   1. Marinate salmon in lemon juice, garlic, and olive oil for 30 minutes.
   2. Preheat the grill to medium heat.
   3. Place salmon on the grill, and season with salt, pepper, and dill.
   4. Grill for 4-5 minutes per side.
   5. Serve with lemon slices.

- Time: 40 minutes

   - Nutritional Information: Salmon is rich in omega-3 fatty acids and provides a good amount of protein.

2. **Herb-Roasted Chicken Breast**

- Ingredients:
- 4 boneless chicken breasts
- 2 tbsp olive oil
- 1 tsp rosemary
- 1 tsp thyme
- 1 tsp oregano
- Salt and pepper to taste

- Instructions:

1. Preheat the oven to 375°F (190°C).
2. Rub chicken with olive oil and herbs.
3. Season with salt and pepper.
4. Roast for 25-30 minutes until cooked through.
5. Let rest before slicing.

- Time: 35 minutes
- Nutritional Information: Chicken breast is a lean protein source and the herbs add flavor without extra calories.

3. **Beef and Broccoli Stir-Fry**
- Ingredients:
- 1 lb beef strips
- 2 cups broccoli florets
- 1 onion, sliced
- 2 tbsp coconut aminos (a soy sauce alternative)
- 1 tbsp sesame oil
- 1 tbsp ginger, grated
- 1 garlic clove, minced

- Instructions:

1. Heat sesame oil in a wok over high heat.

2. Add beef and stir-fry until browned.
3. Add broccoli and onion, and cook until tender.
4. Stir in coconut aminos, ginger, and garlic.
5. Cook for an additional 2 minutes.

- Time: 20 minutes

- Nutritional Information: Beef provides iron and zinc, while broccoli is high in fiber and vitamin C.

4. **Lentil and Spinach Curry**

- Ingredients:
- 1 cup lentils
- 2 cups spinach
- 1 onion, diced
- 2 tomatoes, diced
- 1 tbsp curry powder
- 1 tsp cumin
- 1 tsp turmeric
- 2 cups vegetable broth

- Instructions:

1. Sauté onion in a pot until translucent.
2. Add spices and tomatoes, cook for 2 minutes.
3. Pour in lentils and broth, and bring to a boil.
4. Simmer until lentils are tender.
5. Stir in spinach until wilted.

- Time: 45 minutes

- Nutritional Information: Lentils are a great plant-based protein and high in fiber.

5. **Turkey and Sweet Potato Skillet**

- Ingredients:
- 1 lb ground turkey
- 1 large sweet potato, cubed
- 1 bell pepper, diced
- 1 onion, diced
- 1 tsp paprika
- 1 tsp garlic powder
- Salt and pepper to taste

- Instructions:

1. Brown turkey in a skillet, and set aside.
2. In the same skillet, add sweet potatoes and cook until soft.
3. Add bell pepper and onion, and cook until tender.
4. Return turkey to skillet and season with spices.
5. Cook until everything is heated through.

- Time: 30 minutes
- Nutritional Information: Turkey is a lean source of protein, and sweet potatoes are rich in beta-carotene.

Vegetable-Centric Dishes

1. Kale and Roasted Vegetable Quinoa Bowl
- Ingredients:
- 1 cup quinoa
- 2 cups kale, chopped
- 1 sweet potato, cubed
- 1 red bell pepper, sliced
- 1 zucchini, sliced
- 2 tbsp olive oil
- Salt and pepper to taste

- Instructions:

    1. Cook quinoa as per package instructions.
    2. Toss vegetables in olive oil, salt, and pepper.
    3. Roast in a 400°F oven for 25 minutes.
    4. Mix roasted veggies with cooked quinoa and kale.

- Time: 40 minutes
  - Nutritional Information: Quinoa is a complete protein, and kale is rich in vitamins A, C, and K.

2. **Stuffed Acorn Squash**
   - Ingredients:
   - 2 acorn squash, halved and seeded
   - 1 cup brown rice, cooked
   - 1/2 cup cranberries
   - 1/4 cup pecans, chopped
   - 1/4 cup parsley, chopped
   - 2 tbsp olive oil
   - Salt and pepper to taste

- Instructions:

    1. Roast acorn squash at 375°F until tender, about 30 minutes.
    2. Mix brown rice with cranberries, pecans, and parsley.
    3. Fill squash halves with the rice mixture.
    4. Drizzle with olive oil and season.

- Time: 45 minutes
  - Nutritional Information: High in fiber and antioxidants.

3. **Broccoli and Chickpea Stir-Fry**
   - Ingredients:

- 2 cups broccoli florets
- 1 can chickpeas, drained and rinsed
- 1 onion, sliced
- 2 garlic cloves, minced
- 2 tbsp coconut aminos
- 1 tbsp sesame oil
- Salt and pepper to taste

- Instructions:

1. Heat sesame oil in a pan.
2. Sauté onion and garlic until fragrant.
3. Add broccoli and chickpeas, and cook until tender.
4. Stir in coconut aminos, and season with salt and pepper.

- Time: 20 minutes
- Nutritional Information: Chickpeas are a good source of plant-based protein and fiber.

4. **Spinach and Mushroom Polenta**
   - Ingredients:
   - 1 cup polenta
   - 4 cups water or vegetable broth
   - 2 cups spinach
   - 1 cup mushrooms, sliced
   - 2 tbsp olive oil
   - Salt and pepper to taste

- Instructions:

1. Cook polenta in water or broth as per package instructions.
2. In a separate pan, sauté mushrooms in olive oil.
3. Add spinach until wilted.

4. Serve mushroom and spinach over polenta.

- Time: 30 minutes
   - Nutritional Information: Polenta is gluten-free and a good source of carbohydrates.

5. **Eggplant and Tomato Bake**
   - Ingredients:
   - 1 large eggplant, sliced
   - 2 cups tomatoes, diced
   - 1 onion, diced
   - 3 garlic cloves, minced
   - 1/4 cup fresh basil, chopped
   - 2 tbsp olive oil
   - Salt and pepper to taste

- Instructions:

   1. Layer eggplant slices in a baking dish.
   2. Sauté onion and garlic in olive oil, add tomatoes and basil.
   3. Pour tomato mixture over eggplant.
   4. Bake at 350°F for 30 minutes.

- Time: 45 minutes
   - Nutritional Information: Eggplant is low in calories and high in fiber.

These dishes are packed with vegetables that provide essential nutrients without aggravating Hashimoto's symptoms. They are free from gluten and dairy, aligning with dietary recommendations for Hashimoto's.

Chapter 6: Snacks and Sides

Quick and Easy Snack Ideas

1. **Avocado and Turkey Roll-Ups**
   - Ingredients: Sliced turkey breast, avocado slices
   - Instructions: Lay out turkey slices, place avocado on top, roll them up.
   - Time: 5 minutes
   - Nutritional Information: High in protein and healthy fats.

2. **Carrot and Hummus Dip**
   - Ingredients: Carrot sticks, hummus
   - Instructions: Dip carrot sticks into hummus.
   - Time: 2 minutes
   - Nutritional Information: Rich in fiber and plant-based protein.

3. **Almond Butter Celery Sticks**
   - Ingredients: Celery sticks, almond butter
   - Instructions: Spread almond butter on celery sticks.
   - Time: 5 minutes
   - Nutritional Information: Good source of healthy fats and vitamins.

4. Coconut Yogurt with Berries
   - Ingredients: Coconut yogurt, mixed berries
   - Instructions: Top coconut yogurt with fresh berries.
   - Time: 2 minutes
   - Nutritional Information: Dairy-free, rich in probiotics and antioxidants.

5. Chia Seed Pudding
   - Ingredients: Chia seeds, almond milk, honey
   - Instructions: Mix chia seeds with almond milk, let sit until thickened, and sweeten with honey.
   - Time: Overnight (prep time: 5 minutes)
   - Nutritional Information: High in omega-3 fatty acids and fiber.

6. Cucumber and Smoked Salmon
   - Ingredients: Cucumber slices, smoked salmon
   - Instructions: Top cucumber slices with smoked salmon.
   - Time: 5 minutes
   - Nutritional Information: Source of protein and essential fatty acids.

7. Baked Kale Chips
   - Ingredients: Kale leaves, olive oil, salt
   - Instructions: Toss kale in olive oil, bake until crispy, season with salt.
   - Time: 15 minutes
   - Nutritional Information: Low calorie, high in vitamins A, C, and K.

8. Brazil Nuts
   - Ingredients: Brazil nuts
   - Instructions: Consume a small handful of Brazil nuts.
   - Time: 1 minute
   - Nutritional Information: Selenium-rich, supports thyroid function.

9. Pumpkin Seed Trail Mix
   - Ingredients: Pumpkin seeds, sunflower seeds, unsweetened coconut flakes

- Instructions: Mix ingredients.
- Time: 2 minutes
- Nutritional Information: Magnesium and zinc-rich, energy-boosting.

10. **Green Smoothie**
    - Ingredients: Spinach, banana, almond milk, flaxseeds
    - Instructions: Blend all ingredients until smooth.
    - Time: 5 minutes
    - Nutritional Information: Nutrient-dense, high in fiber and vitamins.

These snacks are designed to be simple and thyroid-friendly, providing a balance of nutrients without common Hashimoto's triggers.

Side Dishes to Complement Any Meal

1. **Roasted Brussels Sprouts with Balsamic Glaze**
    - Ingredients:
    - 1 lb Brussels sprouts, halved
    - 2 tbsp olive oil
    - Salt and pepper to taste
    - 2 tbsp balsamic vinegar

- Instructions:

    1. Toss Brussels sprouts with olive oil, salt, and pepper.
    2. Roast at 400°F for 20-25 minutes until caramelized.
    3. Drizzle with balsamic glaze before serving.

- Time: 30 minutes
    - Nutritional Information: Brussels sprouts are high in fiber and vitamins K and C.

2. **Cauliflower Rice Pilaf**

- Ingredients:
- 1 head cauliflower, riced
- 1 onion, diced
- 2 cloves garlic, minced
- 2 tbsp olive oil
- 1/4 cup chopped parsley
- Salt and pepper to taste

- Instructions:

1. Sauté onion and garlic in olive oil until translucent.
2. Add cauliflower rice, cook for 5-7 minutes.
3. Stir in parsley, and season with salt and pepper.

- Time: 15 minutes
- Nutritional Information: Cauliflower is a low-carb alternative to grains and rich in antioxidants.

3. **Garlic Green Beans**
- Ingredients:
- 1 lb green beans, trimmed
- 3 cloves garlic, minced
- 2 tbsp olive oil
- Salt and pepper to taste

- Instructions:

1. Blanch green beans in boiling water for 3 minutes.
2. Sauté garlic in olive oil until fragrant.
3. Add green beans, sauté for 2-3 minutes.
4. Season with salt and pepper.

- Time: 10 minutes

- Nutritional Information: Green beans are a good source of fiber, vitamin C, and folate.

4. Baked Spiced Sweet Potato Wedges

- Ingredients:
- 2 large sweet potatoes, cut into wedges
- 2 tbsp olive oil
- 1 tsp paprika
- 1/2 tsp cinnamon
- Salt to taste

- Instructions:

1. Toss sweet potato wedges with olive oil, paprika, cinnamon, and salt.
2. Bake at 375°F for 25-30 minutes until tender.

- Time: 35 minutes
- Nutritional Information: Sweet potatoes are high in beta-carotene and fiber

5. Zucchini Noodle Salad

- Ingredients:
- 2 zucchinis, spiralized
- 1/2 cup cherry tomatoes, halved
- 1/4 cup olives, sliced
- 1/4 cup red onion, thinly sliced
- 2 tbsp olive oil
- 1 tbsp lemon juice
- Salt and pepper to taste

- Instructions:

1. Combine zucchini noodles, tomatoes, olives, and onion in a bowl.

2. Whisk together olive oil and lemon juice, and pour over the salad.

3. Toss everything together, and season with salt and pepper.

- Time: 10 minutes

- Nutritional Information: Zucchini is low in calories and a good source of vitamin A.

Dips and Spreads

Here are five dips and spreads that are suitable for a Hashimoto's diet, which generally avoids gluten, dairy, and soy:

1. **Guacamole**
- Ingredients:
- 2 ripe avocados
- 1 small onion, finely chopped
- 1 tomato, diced
- 1 lime, juiced
- 1 clove garlic, minced
- Cilantro, chopped (optional)
- Salt and pepper to taste

- Instructions:

1. Mash the avocados in a bowl.

2. Mix in onion, tomato, lime juice, and garlic.

3. Add cilantro if desired, season with salt and pepper.

- Time: 10 minutes

- Nutritional Information: Avocados are rich in healthy fats and fiber.

2. **Roasted Red Pepper Hummus**
- Ingredients:
- 1 can chickpeas, drained and rinsed

  - 1 roasted red pepper
  - 2 tbsp tahini
  - 2 tbsp olive oil
  - 1 lemon, juiced
  - 1 clove garlic
  - Salt to taste

- Instructions:

  1. Blend all ingredients until smooth.
  2. Adjust seasoning as needed.

- Time: 5 minutes
  - Nutritional Information: Chickpeas provide protein and fiber, while red peppers are high in vitamin C.

3. **Baba Ganoush**
   - Ingredients:
   - 1 large eggplant
   - 2 cloves garlic
   - 2 tbsp tahini
   - 1 lemon, juiced
   - 2 tbsp olive oil
   - Salt and smoked paprika to taste

- Instructions:

  1. Roast the eggplant until tender.
  2. Scoop out the flesh and blend with garlic, tahini, lemon juice, and olive oil.
  3. Season with salt and smoked paprika.

- Time: 45 minutes (including roasting time)

- Nutritional Information: Eggplant is a good source of fiber and antioxidants.

4. **Pumpkin Seed Pesto**
   - Ingredients:
   - 1 cup pumpkin seeds, toasted
   - 2 cups fresh basil leaves
   - 2 cloves garlic
   - 1/2 cup olive oil
   - Salt to taste

- Instructions:

   1. Blend pumpkin seeds, basil, and garlic in a food processor.
   2. Slowly add olive oil until desired consistency is reached.
   3. Season with salt.

- Time: 10 minutes
   - Nutritional Information: Pumpkin seeds are rich in magnesium and zinc, which are beneficial for thyroid health.

5. **Sunflower Seed Butter**
   - Ingredients:
   - 2 cups sunflower seeds, toasted
   - 2 tbsp coconut oil
   - 1 tbsp honey (optional)
   - Salt to taste

- Instructions:

   1. Blend sunflower seeds in a food processor until creamy.
   2. Add coconut oil and honey if using, and blend until smooth.
   3. Season with salt.

- Time: 15 minutes

   - Nutritional Information: Sunflower seeds are a great source of vitamin E and selenium.

These dips and spreads are designed to be easy to make and thyroid-friendly, providing a variety of flavors and nutrients without common Hashimoto's triggers.

Chapter 7: Desserts and Treats

Guilt-Free Sweet Treats

Guilt-free sweet treats that are suitable for Hashimoto's diet:

1. **Chocolate-Covered Almonds**
   - Ingredients:
- 1 cup raw almonds
- 1/2 cup dark chocolate chips (at least 70% cacao)
- Instructions:

1. Melt the chocolate chips in a double boiler or microwave.
2. Dip the almonds in the melted chocolate and place them on a parchment-lined tray.
3. Refrigerate until the chocolate sets.

- Time: 15 minutes
   - Nutritional Information: Almonds are rich in healthy fats and protein, while dark chocolate is high in antioxidants.

2. **Peanut Butter and Cacao Nib Bites**
   - Ingredients:

- 1/2 cup natural peanut butter
- 1/4 cup cacao nibs
- 1/4 cup coconut flour
- Instructions:

1. Mix peanut butter and coconut flour until well combined.
2. Stir in cacao nibs.
3. Roll the mixture into small balls and refrigerate.

- Time: 20 minutes
- Nutritional Information: Peanut butter provides protein and healthy fats, and cacao nibs offer a chocolate flavor without added sugar.

3. **Fruit Drizzled with Honey**
   - Ingredients:
   - Your choice of diced fruit (e.g., apples, pears, bananas)
   - Honey for drizzling
   - Instructions:

1. Arrange diced fruit on a plate.
2. Lightly drizzle with honey.

- Time: 5 minutes
- Nutritional Information: Fruits provide essential vitamins and fiber, and honey adds natural sweetness.

4. **Coconut Yogurt with Mixed Berries**
   - Ingredients:
   - 1 cup unsweetened coconut yogurt
   - 1/2 cup mixed berries (strawberries, blueberries, raspberries)
   - Instructions:

1. Spoon coconut yogurt into a bowl.

2. Top with mixed berries.

- Time: 2 minutes
   - Nutritional Information: Coconut yogurt is a dairy-free probiotic source, and berries are low in sugar and high in antioxidants.

5. **Banana and Almond Butter Toast**
   - Ingredients:
   - 1 slice of gluten-free bread, toasted
   - 1 tablespoon almond butter
   - 1/2 banana, sliced
   - Instructions:

   1. Spread almond butter on the toasted bread.
   2. Arrange banana slices on top.

- Time: 5 minutes
   - Nutritional Information: This treat is a good source of healthy fats from almond butter and potassium from bananas.

These treats are designed to satisfy your sweet tooth without compromising Hashimoto's diet. They are free from gluten, dairy, and refined sugars, which can be inflammatory.

Baked Goods Made with Alternative Flours

1. **Almond Flour Banana Bread**
   - Ingredients:
   - 2 cups almond flour
   - 3 ripe bananas, mashed
   - 2 eggs
   - 1/4 cup honey
   - 1 tsp baking soda

- 1/2 tsp salt
- 1 tsp vanilla extract

- Instructions:

1. Preheat the oven to 350°F (175°C).
2. Mix all ingredients until well combined.
3. Pour into a greased loaf pan.
4. Bake for 45-50 minutes or until a toothpick comes out clean.

- Time: 1 hour
  - Nutritional Information: Almond flour is gluten-free and rich in protein and healthy fats.

2. **Coconut Flour Chocolate Chip Cookies**
   - Ingredients:
   - 3/4 cup coconut flour
   - 1/2 cup coconut oil, melted
   - 1/2 cup maple syrup
   - 2 eggs
   - 1/2 tsp baking soda
   - 1/4 tsp salt
   - 1/2 cup dark chocolate chips

- Instructions:

1. Preheat the oven to 350°F (175°C).
2. Combine coconut flour, coconut oil, maple syrup, eggs, baking soda, and salt.
3. Fold in chocolate chips.
4. Drop spoonfuls onto a baking sheet and flatten slightly.
5. Bake for 12-15 minutes.

- Time: 30 minutes
  - Nutritional Information: Coconut flour is high in fiber and makes a great low-carb alternative to wheat flour.

3. **Buckwheat Pancakes**
   - Ingredients:
   - 1 cup buckwheat flour
   - 1 tbsp sugar
   - 1 tsp baking powder
   - 1/2 tsp salt
   - 1 egg
   - 1 cup almond milk
   - 2 tbsp melted coconut oil

- Instructions:

   1. Mix the dry ingredients.
   2. In another bowl, whisk the wet ingredients.
   3. Combine both mixtures until smooth.
   4. Pour batter onto a hot griddle and cook until bubbles form, then flip.

- Time: 20 minutes
  - Nutritional Information: Buckwheat is gluten-free and contains a good amount of protein and fiber.

4. **Quinoa Flour Muffins**
   - Ingredients:
   - 2 cups quinoa flour
   - 1/2 cup applesauce
   - 1/4 cup olive oil
   - 1/2 cup honey
   - 2 eggs
   - 1 tsp baking powder

- 1/2 tsp salt
- 1 cup blueberries

- Instructions:

  1. Preheat the oven to 350°F (175°C).
  2. Mix all ingredients except blueberries until well combined.
  3. Gently fold in blueberries.
  4. Spoon into muffin tins and bake for 20-25 minutes.

- Time: 45 minutes
  - Nutritional Information: Quinoa flour is a complete protein source and is rich in amino acids.

5. **Oat Flour Apple Crisp**
  - Ingredients:
  - 2 cups oat flour
  - 4 apples, peeled and sliced
  - 1/2 cup coconut sugar
  - 1/2 cup unsalted butter, melted
  - 1 tsp cinnamon
  - Pinch of salt

- Instructions:

  1. Preheat the oven to 375°F (190°C).
  2. Layer apple slices in a baking dish.
  3. Mix oat flour, coconut sugar, melted butter, cinnamon, and salt until crumbly.
  4. Sprinkle over the apples and bake for 30-35 minutes.

- Time: 45 minutes
  - Nutritional Information: Oat flour is a heart-healthy option high in

soluble fiber.

These recipes provide delicious alternatives to traditional baked goods, using flours that are more suitable for Hashimoto's Thyroiditis. They are gluten-free and use natural sweeteners, aligning with dietary recommendations for Hashimoto's.

Frozen Desserts

1. Mixed Berry Sorbet
   - Ingredients:
   - 1 1/4 cups frozen mixed berries (strawberries, blueberries, raspberries)
   - 1 small frozen banana
   - 1/2 cup unsweetened coconut, almond, or cashew milk
   - 1 tablespoon maple syrup

- Instructions:

   1. Blend all ingredients until smooth.
   2. Freeze the mixture until set, about 2 hours.
   3. Serve chilled.

- Time: 2 hours 5 minutes
   - Nutritional Information: Rich in antioxidants and naturally sweetened.

2. Coconut Chocolate Bars
   - Ingredients:
   - 2 cups shredded unsweetened coconut
   - 1/2 cup coconut oil, melted
   - 1/4 cup honey
   - 1/2 cup dark chocolate, melted

- Instructions:

1. Mix coconut, coconut oil, and honey.
2. Press into a lined baking dish and freeze until firm.
3. Drizzle with melted dark chocolate and return to the freezer.
4. Cut into bars once set.

- Time: 1 hour
   - Nutritional Information: Free from dairy and gluten, with healthy fats from coconut.

3. **Pineapple Mango Ice Pops**
   - Ingredients:
   - 2 cups fresh pineapple, chopped
   - 1 cup mango, chopped
   - 1/2 cup water or coconut water

- Instructions:

1. Blend pineapple, mango, and water until smooth.
2. Pour into ice pop molds and freeze until solid.

- Time: 4 hours
   - Nutritional Information: A refreshing treat with no added sugar, rich in vitamins A and C.

4. **Banana Almond Butter Ice Cream**
   - Ingredients:
   - 4 ripe bananas, sliced and frozen
   - 2 tablespoons almond butter
   - 1 teaspoon vanilla extract

- Instructions:

1. Blend frozen bananas until creamy.

2. Add almond butter and vanilla, and blend until mixed.
3. Freeze until desired consistency is reached.

- Time: 2 hours
   - Nutritional Information: Dairy-free and contains potassium and healthy fats.

5. **Avocado Lime Ice Cream**
   - Ingredients:
   - 2 ripe avocados
   - 1/2 cup lime juice
   - 1/4 cup honey
   - 1/2 cup coconut milk

- Instructions:

   1. Blend avocados, lime juice, honey, and coconut milk until smooth.
   2. Freeze in an airtight container until set.

- Time: 4 hours
   - Nutritional Information: Creamy and rich in healthy fats, with a tangy lime flavor.

These frozen desserts are designed to be enjoyable without compromising the dietary restrictions commonly associated with Hashimoto's Hypothyroidism.

Chapter 8: Healing Herbs and Supplements

Herbs that aid thyroid health

1ist of herbs that help in managing thyroid health, along with their possible benefits:

1. Ashwagandha (Withania somnifera).

- Benefits: This adaptogenic herb has been shown to relieve stress and improve thyroid function by modulating hormone levels. It's known for its ability to boost T4 conversion to the more active T3 hormone.

2. Bacopa Monnieri.

- Benefits: Bacopa monnieri, which is commonly used in Ayurvedic medicine, may improve both hypo and hyperthyroidism. Research suggests it may improve cognitive function and control thyroid hormone production.

3. Ginger

- Benefits: Ginger contains anti-inflammatory, antioxidant, and antibacterial properties. It may aid hypothyroidism patients by regulating hormone levels and decreasing inflammation.

4. Holy basil (Ocimum tenuiflorum)

Benefits: Holy basil, also known as tulsi, is an adaptogen that can help the body adapt to stress and balance hormone levels, potentially supporting thyroid health.

5. Lemon Balm

- Benefits: Lemon balm is thought to help regulate an overactive thyroid by lowering thyroid hormone levels. It has relaxing effects and may help with stress-related thyroid issues.

6. Nettle

- Benefits: Nettle contains minerals that may promote thyroid function due to its iodine level. However, it's vital to watch iodine intake as both excess and shortage can impact the thyroid.

7. Black Walnut

- Benefits: Black walnuts contain a lot of iodine and have long been used to help with thyroid function. It may be especially useful in cases of iodine deficiency.

8. Schisandra

Benefits: Schisandra is an adaptogen that can improve liver function and hormonal balance, thereby boosting thyroid health.

9. Maca (Lepidium meyenii).

Benefits: Maca root can balance hormones and support thyroid function.

10. Bladderwrack (fucus vesiculosus)

- Benefits: Bladderwrack is a form of seaweed rich in iodine, which is essential for thyroid health. It is commonly used to treat hypothyroidism caused by low iodine levels.

Supplements For Hashimoto's

Supplements can help manage Hashimoto's Thyroiditis by treating vitamin shortages and promoting thyroid health. Here's a list of supplements that could be useful:

1. Vitamin D

- Benefits: Supports immunological function and may minimize autoimmune activity.

2. Selenium

- Benefits include thyroid hormone production and antioxidant protection, as well as a potential reduction in thyroid antibody levels.

3. Inositol

- Benefits: A form of sugar that can alter insulin and hormones involved with mood and cognition, and may assist improve thyroid function when taken with selenium.

4. Zinc

- Benefits: Supports immunological function and thyroid hormone metabolism.

5. Magnesium

- Benefits: Promotes several enzymatic activities, including those required for thyroid function.

6. Iron

- Benefits: Helps synthesize thyroid hormones and may be inadequate in hypothyroid patients.

7. Dehydroepiandrosterone (DHEA)

- Benefits: A hormone that can boost the immune system and balance other hormones in the body.

8. Black Cumin Seed

- Benefits: May reduce inflammation and boost immunological health.

9. Probiotics

- Benefits: Promote gut health, which enhances immunological function and may indirectly improve thyroid health.

10. L-Glutamine

- Benefits: An amino acid promotes gut lining integrity, avoiding autoimmune reactions.

How to Include Them in Your Diet

When controlling Hashimoto's, there are a few crucial steps to include supplements and herbs in your diet.

1. Consult with a healthcare provider.

They can help decide which supplements may be appropriate for your unique health needs and verify no problems with your current medications or treatments.

2. Identify your needs.

Understand which nutrients you may be lacking and which herbs may benefit your thyroid health. Vitamin D, selenium, zinc, and magnesium are common supplements for Hashimoto's disease. Adaptogenic herbs, such as ashwagandha and holy basil, can balance hormones and reduce stress.

3. Quality Matters:

Select high-quality vitamins and botanicals. Look for recognized brands that have undergone third-party testing to assure purity and efficacy.

4. Start slowly:

When introducing new supplements or herbs, begin with a small amount and gradually increase as directed by your healthcare professional. This allows you to monitor your body's response and reduce potential negative effects.

5. Monitor your response:

Keep track of any changes in your symptoms or adverse effects once you start taking vitamins or herbs. This information can help your healthcare practitioner change your regimen as necessary.

6. Dietary integration:

Incorporate herbs into your diet by cooking them or making drinks. For example, you can include ginger in stir-fries or take a cup of lemon balm tea before bed. Supplements can be taken in pill or liquid form with meals unless advised differently by your healthcare provider.

7. Regular Testing:

Schedule regular blood tests to assess your thyroid function and nutrient levels. This can aid in adjusting supplement amounts and ensuring that you are not receiving too much or too little of a specific nutrient.

8. Lifestyle considerations:

Remember that vitamins and herbs are only one component of a holistic approach to Hashimoto's disease management. Maintaining thyroid health requires a balanced diet, frequent exercise, stress management, and proper sleep.

Always remember that, while vitamins and herbs might be beneficial, they should not be used in place of conventional treatments recommended by your healthcare physician. These natural therapies should be used as part of a full treatment plan for Hashimoto's hypothyroidism.

Chapter 9: Meal Planning and Preparation

Tips for batch cooking and food preparation

Batch cooking and food preparation are practices that can change the way you approach meals, making healthy eating more doable and time-efficient. This comprehensive tutorial will help you master the art of batch cooking and food preparation.

Understand Batch Cooking

Batch cooking is the process of preparing big amounts of food at once to be consumed over days or weeks. It's an approach that will save you time, minimize stress, and ensure you always have healthy, cooked meals on hand. The goal is to cook once or twice a week and eat several times, which reduces the amount of effort required to produce fresh meals every day.

Benefits of Batch Cooking

- Time Efficiency: Cooking in batches saves time in the kitchen overall. You just have to prepare and clean once, yet the effort yields numerous meals.

- Cost-Effective: Purchasing ingredients in bulk often results in cost savings. Furthermore, you are less likely to dine out or order takeout, which can be more expensive than home-cooked meals.

- Healthier Eating: Keeping ready-to-eat healthy meals in your fridge or freezer makes you less likely to reach for unhealthy snacks or fast food.

- Reduced Food Waste: Planning your meals and cooking in batches increases the likelihood that you will use all of the ingredients you purchase, lowering the quantity of food that goes to waste.

Getting started with batch cooking

1. Plan Your Meals: Determine what you want to consume throughout the week. Consider meals that store well and are easy to reheat.
2. Make a Shopping List: Using your food plan, build a shopping list. Stick to it to minimize impulse purchases and make sure you have what you need.
3. Set aside time: Pick a day when you have a few hours to devote to cooking. Many folks find that weekends work best.
4. Wash, chop, and prepare your ingredients. This makes the cooking process run more smoothly and quickly.
5. Cook in batches: Prepare huge amounts of food that may be divided into individual servings. Soups, stews, casseroles, and stir-fries are excellent choices.
6. Store your meals in sealed containers. Label them with the date and contents to keep track of what you own.
7. Reheat and Enjoy: Simply reheat your prepared meals throughout the week. This saves time and guarantees that you have a healthy supper ready to go.

Food Preparation Tips

- Invest in Quality Containers: Proper storage containers are vital for keeping food fresh. Consider using glass or BPA-free plastic containers with tight-fitting lids.

- Cook Versatile Ingredients: Prepare ingredients that can be utilized in a variety of meals. For example, roast a tray of mixed veggies that may be used in salads, wraps, or as a side dish.

- Use the Freezer: Not all meals have to be consumed within a week. Freeze portions for later use, which can be a lifesaver on especially hectic days.

- Season Wisely: When cooking items rather than complete meals, season gently. This allows you to adjust the flavor of your meals as you assemble them.

- Keep It Simple: Don't complicate your meal preparation. Simple, healthful ingredients can be just as tasty and much more convenient to prepare in large amounts.

Batch Cooking Techniques

- Double or treble Recipes: To cook, simply double or treble the recipe. This is one of the simplest ways to batch cook without having to learn a new recipe.

- Theme Your Days: Some people find it useful to theme their cooking days (for example, Meatless Monday, Taco Tuesday) to add diversity and structure to their meal planning.

- Cook Once, Eat Twice: Make a larger serving for dinner and save the leftovers for lunch the next day.

- Assembly Line Style: Set up an assembly line for chores like filling containers or putting together wraps. This can speed up and improve the process's efficiency.

Common Mistakes To Avoid

- Overcomplicating Recipes: Stick with recipes you're familiar with. Trying too many new or complicated dishes at once might be exhausting.

- Failing to plan for variety: Eating the same meal repeatedly can become monotonous. Plan for a variety of flavors and textures to keep things interesting.

- Neglecting to Label: Always label your containers. It is easy to forget what is within, especially after it has been frozen.

- Ignoring Food Safety: Be aware of how long food can be safely stored. Use up older meals first, and follow correct freezing and thawing procedures.

Conclusion

Batch cooking and food preparation are about more than just saving time; they're also about developing long-term, healthy eating habits. With a little forethought and some basic procedures, you may enjoy fresh meals that suit your lifestyle and interests. Remember, the secret to successful batch cooking is to start simply, be consistent, and figure out what works best for you. Happy cooking!

Shopping Lists and Storage Solutions

When creating a shopping list for Hashimoto's diet, prioritize complete, nutrient-dense foods that promote thyroid health. Here's a general outline of what you could include:

Shopping List for the Hashimoto's Diet

- Animal protein options include chicken, turkey, and fish such as salmon and cod.

- Non-starchy vegetables include artichokes, asparagus, and broccoli, as well as leafy greens like kale and spinach.

- Fruits: Low-sugar selections include berries, apples, and citrus fruits.

- Healthy fats include avocado, almonds, seeds, and extra virgin olive oil.

- Gluten-free whole grains include brown rice, quinoa, and rolled oats.

- Dairy and non-dairy substitutes include almond milk, coconut yogurt, and goat cheese.

- Beans and legumes include lentils, chickpeas, and black beans.

- Ingredients include apple cider vinegar, basil, turmeric, and honey.

Storage options for batch cooking

- Airtight Containers: Use high-quality containers to keep food fresh. Glass containers, such as Pyrex, and BPA-free plastic products are excellent choices.

- Stay organized by clearly labeling each container with contents and preparation date.

- Freezer Bags: Use durable freezer bags to prevent freezer burn and conserve space.

- Nesting bowls can conserve cupboard space and are microwave and freezer safe.

- Reusable silicone bags are eco-friendly and ideal for storing snacks or small meal portions.

Remember that adequate organization and storage are essential for efficient meal preparation and batch cooking. By tailoring your shopping list to Hashimoto's diet and using smart storage options, you can ensure that your meals stay fresh and delicious all week. Happy cooking and healthy eating.

Stress Management Techniques

Stress management is critical for people living with Hashimoto's disease because it can have a significant impact on thyroid function. Here are some effective stress management techniques tailored for people with Hashimoto's.

1. Mindfulness Meditation entails being completely present in the moment and accepting it without judgment. Meditation can reduce stress by enhancing your response to stressors.
2. Deep Breathing Exercises: Deep breathing stimulates the body's relaxation response. Diaphragmatic breathing, which focuses on filling the lungs, can be especially beneficial.
3. Yoga uses physical postures, breathing exercises, and meditation to promote relaxation and reduce stress.
4. Regular exercise can help reduce stress hormones and improve mood. Gentle activities such as walking or swimming can be beneficial.
5. Getting 7-9 hours of quality sleep per night can regulate stress hormones and improve overall health.
6. A well-balanced diet that promotes thyroid health can also help with stress management. Choose whole foods over processed and sugary options.
7. Time Management: Organizing your schedule and setting achievable goals can help alleviate the stress of feeling overwhelmed.
8. Social Support: Connecting with friends, family, or support groups can help you feel less isolated.
9. Professional Help: Speaking with a therapist or counselor can sometimes

help you develop personalized stress management strategies.

10. Other effective relaxation techniques include progressive muscle relaxation, guided imagery, and aromatherapy.

Remember that what works for one person may not work for another, so identify the techniques that work best for you and incorporate them into your daily routine. Consistency is essential for managing stress and promoting thyroid health

.

Connecting with Others in the Hashimoto's Journey

Connecting with others who are on the same Hashimoto's journey can be extremely beneficial and enlightening. Here are a few ways to build connections:

1. Join Support Groups: Hashimoto's patients can share their experiences and advice through various online platforms, such as Facebook groups and forums.
2. Attend Workshops and Seminars: Look for local or virtual events focusing on thyroid health and Hashimoto's disease to connect with others in similar situations.
3. Follow blogs and websites: Many professionals and patients share their tales and tips online, creating a sense of community and connection.
4. Participate in Local Health Fairs: These events provide an excellent opportunity to meet with healthcare practitioners and people living with Hashimoto's.
5. Volunteer: Giving your time to connected health groups can help you connect with others who understand what you're going through.

Conclusion

As we near the end of our Hashimoto's diet recipes cookbook, remember that each dish you've discovered is more than simply a meal; it's a step toward better health and well-being. This collection of dishes is intended to nourish your body, support your thyroid, and bring joy into your kitchen. The journey with Hashimoto's is profoundly personal, and what works for one person may not work for another, but the goal of this cookbook is to provide you with the tools you need to experiment and discover what works best for your health.

Accept the process of learning about your body, identifying your specific needs, and enjoying tiny triumphs on your path to wellness. May this cookbook be a reliable friend on your path, providing comfort in the form of delicious, nourishing meals that adhere to the principles of Hashimoto's diet. Here's to achieving balance, enjoying flavors, and surviving with Hashimoto's.

www.ingramcontent.com/pod-product-compliance
Lightning Source LLC
Chambersburg PA
CBHW050819250726
48653CB00006B/2306